CHOCOLATE
DELIGHT

CHOCOLATE
DELIGHT

Become a Chocolate Expert

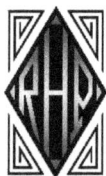

Roland Duvall

Table of Contents

1. Introduction

We are really excited to have you here with us with our chocolate appreciation book, because the thing I'm really passionate about is sharing the world's best chocolate with you. And as we go through today, you're going to learn what the world's best chocolate is.

I have some of it here as some examples. And of course, we'll go through some tasting. And one of the how I got into this and what I want to take you through is the experience that I had some years ago, maybe about 10 years ago.

I went to a chocolate appreciation class. Now, before that, I consider myself a chocoholic. I ate chocolate every day. I still do and thought I knew everything about chocolate.

And I went to this master class where I learned about these exceptional brands I've never heard of before, had no idea about.

And it blew my mind and opened my eyes that there's so much more to chocolate than what I, I knew. And what I realized through that is that I wasn't really a chocoholic. I was a Cadbury acholic or maybe a sugar acholic.

And since then, I've been on a real journey of learning about chocolate and sharing this passion with others. So, as we go through today, we're going to talk about all the different facets of chocolate that you've probably never even thought about before. And at the end of it, you're going to be your very own chocolate expert. So, enjoy the journey with me.

2. What is the world's best chocolate?

So, the next topic we're going to talk about for you to become a chocolate expert is ethics. It's by far the most negative, I guess, a topic that we're going to talk about.

But we're going to finish on a good note, because by the end of this, you'll know how to not only find the world's best chocolate, but the most ethical as well, which is really important because the chocolate industry is plagued with problems around ethics, particularly with the chocolate that comes out of West Africa, so that Ghana and Ivory Coast that we've been talking about and in those countries of Ghana and the Ivory Coast, you've got endemic problems that for the most part probably result in, at best poverty and at worst, much worse things such as forced labor, child labor and even death.

So, if we talk about poverty, there has been a global poverty line set at one dollar ninety US and anything anyone earning that up below that is considered to be living in poverty. If you look at what Cacao workers in Ghana and the Ivory Coast are earning, they're earning a median wage of between 75 cents and around 50 cents a day, so well below that poverty line. So, we've already got a huge issue with poverty.

These farmers and these workers aren't earning enough to live off. Secondly, we then get into issues around forced labor, which is a huge problem we have in the adult population working in Ghana and the Ivory Coast, up to thirteen thousand adults who have experienced forced labor.

And there's the potential that that figure is actually quite a bit higher. One of the problems we have is as consumers demand cheaper prices, as the market changes and prices come down, that puts more pressure on farmers to run at a certain cost.

And it means they're more likely to use forced labor. It also means they're more likely to use child labor. This is a really big problem in Ghana and the Ivory Coast and in those countries at the moment, you've got around two million children working in that industry and we're talking about quite young children.

So, in the Ivory Coast, for example, 41 percent of those children working in the industry are between the ages of 10 and 11. So, we're talking very young children. All of those children are exposed to hazardous workplaces, whether it's shop items with the machetes used to cut the Cacao pods, agrochemicals, heavy loads, et cetera. In addition of those children, there's a significantly high number who are forced labor as well, and they're being forced by somebody other than their parents.

So, when we talk about ethics, there's so much that we can talk about and there's examples that we can give. But I think it's important for us to move on and recognize what places, countries and what companies are doing great things with ethics because they exist out there, which is the wonderful thing. So, as we mentioned at the start, the bulk of the problems from come from Ghana and the Ivory Coast.

So, No one, when you're getting your chocolate from somewhere other than that, the ethics inherently go up quite quickly. When you look at companies that iStock and that are the world's best, the great news is I've got an example here of Valrhona that they typically have exceptional ethics around them, the best of the best. And what's interesting is they might not have a label on them.

So, all the chocolate iStock like this Valrhona one, for example, they position themselves in the market as a flavor chocolate, because if you remember back to what's the world's best chocolate, it's an amazing bean with amazing processing. So that's what they're all about. But each one of these companies wants to and has to have the highest of ethics. Otherwise, they can't secure those beans.

So don't believe the labels. Fairtrade, for example, isn't enough. There's also a lot of controversy about fair trade, whether it actually delivers real benefits to farmers. If you jump online, you can find out some more on that. But jump on a company's website, for example, this particular chocolate Manjiro, which comes from

Madagascar, amazing chocolate producing come true.

If you jump in line with Valrhona, you will find a video of this particular plantation where you can see what's happening. You can see that they're building new housing for the workers. You can see the programs empowering women and so forth, because this is what you're looking for. Jump on a chocolate producers' website and they should have really clear evidence of what they're doing.

They should be doing more than just paying a fair price. They because that's not enough to pay just a fair price. They should be community programs that are building schools that are teaching business skills, that are supporting biodiversity of crops, that are supporting women in those communities. And they should be trading directly with the farmers or with the co-op that's running that particular plantation.

So, things to look for, look for those programs, look for direct trade, look for transparency. If a chocolate company can tell you where they're coming from, that's transparency. That's what you want for Rona, for example, has just. Certified as a big corporation, which companies that are leading economic change through not doing any harm to anyone else and not doing any harm to the environment. So, look for external certification. What you don't want to buy when it comes to ethics is sort of a chocolate that is certified by the company. If you look at Cadbury, for example, which is an obvious chocolate to talk about, at some point, they have their own Catalo life program, but there is no external auditing of that program. There is no transparency. There's nothing to tell us that that's actually effective. So, scratch the surface, find the evidence. Chocolate that's made from amazing beans is typically going to be ethical and enjoy your chocolate milk free.

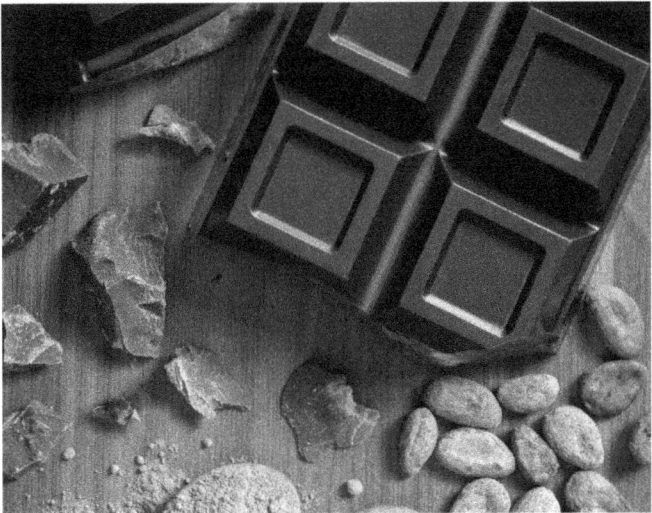

3. Ethical Chocolate

So, the next topic we're going to talk about for you to become a chocolate expert is ethics. It's by far the most negative, I guess, a topic that we're going to talk about.

But we're going to finish on a good note, because by the end of this, you'll know how to not only find the world's best chocolate, but the most ethical as well, which is really important because the chocolate industry is plagued with problems around ethics, particularly with the chocolate that comes out of West Africa, so that Ghana and Ivory Coast that we've been talking about and in those countries of Ghana and the Ivory Coast, you've got endemic problems that for the most part probably result in, at best poverty and at worst, much worse things such as forced labor, child labor and even death.

So, if we talk about poverty, there has been a global poverty line set at one dollar ninety US and anything anyone earning that up below that is considered to be living in poverty. If you look at what Cacao workers in Ghana and the Ivory Coast are earning, they're earning a median wage of between 75 cents and around 50 cents a day, so well below that poverty line. So, we've already got a huge issue with poverty.

These farmers and these workers aren't earning enough to live off. Secondly, we then get into issues around forced labor, which is a huge problem we have in the adult population working in Ghana and the Ivory Coast, up to thirteen thousand adults who have experienced forced labor.

And there's the potential that that figure is actually quite a bit higher. One of the problems we have is as consumers demand cheaper prices, as the market changes and prices come down, that puts more pressure on farmers to run at a certain cost. And it means they're more likely to use forced labor. It also means they're more likely to use child labor.

This is a really big problem in Ghana and the Ivory Coast and in those countries at the moment, you've got around two million children working in that industry and we're talking about quite young children. So, in the Ivory Coast, for example, 41 percent of those children working in the industry are between the ages of 10 and 11.

So, we're talking very young children. All of those children are exposed to hazardous workplaces, whether it's shop items with the machetes used to cut the Cacao pods, agrochemicals, heavy loads, et cetera. In addition of those children, there's a significantly high number who are forced labor as well, and they're being forced by somebody other than their parents. So, when we talk about ethics, there's so much that we can talk about and there's examples that we can give.

But I think it's important for us to move on and recognize what places, countries and what companies are doing great things with ethics because they exist out there, which is the wonderful thing.

So, as we mentioned at the start, the bulk of the problems from come from Ghana and the Ivory Coast. So, No one, when you're getting your chocolate from somewhere other than that, the ethics inherently go up quite quickly.

When you look at companies that iStock and that are the world's best, the great news is I've got an example here of Valrhona that they typically have exceptional ethics around them, the best of the best. And what's interesting is they might not have a label on them.

So, all the chocolate iStock like this Valrhona one, for example, they position themselves in the market as a flavor chocolate, because if you remember back to what's the world's best chocolate, it's an amazing bean with amazing processing.

So that's what they're all about. But each one of these companies wants to and has to have the highest of ethics. Otherwise, they can't secure those beans.

So don't believe the labels. Fairtrade, for example, isn't enough. There's also a lot of controversy about fair trade, whether it actually delivers real benefits to farmers. If you jump online, you can find out some more on that. But jump on a company's website, for example, this particular chocolate Manjiro, which comes from Madagascar, amazing chocolate producing come true.

If you jump in line with Valrhona, you will find a video of this particular plantation where you can see what's happening. You can see that they're building new housing for the workers.

You can see the programs empowering women and so forth, because this is what you're looking for. Jump on a chocolate producers' website and they should have really clear evidence of what they're doing.

They should be doing more than just paying a fair price. They because that's not enough to pay just a fair price. They should be community programs that are building schools that are teaching business skills, that are supporting biodiversity of crops, that are supporting women in those communities.

And they should be trading directly with the farmers or with the co-op that's running that particular plantation.

So, things to look for, look for those programs, look for direct trade, look for transparency. If a chocolate company can tell you where they're coming from, that's transparency. That's what you want for Rona, for example, has just.

Certified as a big corporation, which companies that are leading economic change through not doing any harm to anyone else and not doing any harm to the environment. So, look for external certification. What you don't want to buy when it comes to ethics is sort of a chocolate that is certified by the company.

If you look at Cadbury, for example, which is an obvious chocolate to talk about, at some point, they have their own Catalo life program, but there is no external auditing of that program. There is no transparency.

There's nothing to tell us that that's actually effective. So, scratch the surface, find the evidence. Chocolate that's made from amazing beans is typically going to be ethical and enjoy your chocolate milk free.

The Political Geography of
CHOCOLATE
Global Cocoa Trade Organizations

ORGANIZATIONS
International Cocoa Organization (ICCO)
Alliance of Cocoa Producing Countries (COPAL)

COPAL & ICCO (Exporting)
COPAL Only
ICCO Only (Exporting)
ICCO Only (Importing)

4. The history of chocolate - from the Olmecs to the Aztecs

Your next step into becoming a chocolate expert is to learn a little bit about the history, and you might think that history might think of a European history, but we need to go much further back in time to understand where chocolate comes from.

And what I love about the history of chocolate is we're going to go back to fifteen hundred B.C. to start with to the mix. And from that time to modern day time is this amazing love humans have had with chocolate and with Cacao, which has just transcended all of that time.

This is one commonality that goes through with that. So, we start with the first recorded use of Cacao by humans. We go back to the OMICS who are one of the Mizo American tribes in Central America. They're a little bit mysterious. Our friends, the mix, we don't know too much about them. We know that they invented ballgames. They were the first of the Mizo American societies to start bloodletting, which went to a real fervor in Aztec times with sacrifices.

They built big, colossal heads, these enormous, colossal heads that people can't understand how they built them. And we know from those that physically they looked very different from the Mayans and the Aztecs who followed them.

But they were also the first culture to cultivate Cacao, which is the Cerillo mean. If you remember when we were talking about the different vein types, I mentioned the Cerillo being was the first domesticated Cacao and thought to be the original.

So the Olmec had amazing agricultural skills well before their time and they started growing. How they also gave us the first word that starts to sound like a cow that starts coming through these societies.

And there's the word Krakauer that comes from the Amax. Now, obviously, we've got beans growing economic times and no blocks of chocolate blocks of chocolate came much, much later.

And in fact, a very recent addition to the story about chocolate, the oil mixed with drinking their chocolate, as most of humans have done for the last two and a half thousand, three and a half thousand years.

And they were making a frothy hot chocolate. So even as far back as the Olmec times, what they were doing is they were grinding up the cocoa beans, similar to what we still do today. We still grind cocoa beans and they're all mixing it with various substances and then with water to make a drink.

And they would make it frothy by taking two vessels and pouring it at great height from one to the other. One of the things we know about the Caribbean is its approximately 50 percent cocoa butter and 50 percent Cacao solid.

So, it's actually quite fatty. But when you're having this sequence of pouring going on, that fat is going to turn into a really frothy drink so that we're drinking hot chocolate. It was frothy. It was very ritualized.

So as an average layperson, I probably was never going to be able to drink a cup of cocoa in Olmec times. It was really for priest aristocracy and for rituals. Now we're drinking Cacao back in the Olmec times.

And that's going to continue through when we're talking about chocolate up until well past the Spanish into the English. We're talking about it as a drink, which will continue to elaborate on how it changed over the times.

So got the Olmec starting it with. The mix was followed by the Mayans who were a very advanced civilization again, and they continued the love of bloodletting, and they also continued the love of Cacao. And you see through all those these Mesoamerican societies, you see this combination of ritualized bloodletting and sacrifice and Cacao intersecting. So the Mayans, for example, believed that the gods shed their blood on the Cacao pods, and that's possibly because of the color of the cocoa pods, which are bright reds and purples and so forth.

Again, very much used in rituals very much used by priests and not for the average layperson. The Mayans, however, started to change things a little bit because they started to cultivate chilies. And this whole thing we see about chili and chocolate now is nothing new.

This goes back to the Mayan times. They would they had lots of different ways to drink a cow, but one of the favorite ones was with Chili and Wild Honey. They would drink a cold that would use it in all sorts of ceremonies and also mixing it with a maze, grill and water, which I don't know that that sounds very appetizing.

I think I'll take the Chili and honey version. But what we know most about is how the Aztecs used Cacao, because when we talk about the Aztecs, we're also talking about when the Spanish arrived, and those two different cultures intersected.

So, we know that they still revere it, they really took the love of Cacao on the ritualize love of kickout, a whole other level, the Aztecs took a lot of things to a whole other level, for that matter, including the human sacrifice element. There was a reconsideration of a grand pyramid at the end of the fourteen hundreds, and they were said to be eighty thousand people sacrificed in the Aztec community. And even every year, even aside from that, every year you had thousands of people being human sacrifices. The one good thing about being a human sacrifice during Aztec times is you were given a cocktail pod as part of that ritual.

So that was meant to help you go to the heavens and B, make everything OK for being sacrificed by highly ritualized, destroying a lot of banquets.

There's evidence from the Spanish in their reports that they would mix a particular local seed with the hot chocolate, which was which was red and would make the drink red and it would stay in their mouth completely red.

So, the Spanish always said that it looked like they'd been drinking blood, which just fits with that whole Aztec ethos. But at the time, the only people who could consume Cacao were again with them, but the aristocracy and impro, Montezuma's army.

There's one report that his army would, in fact, have a Kakao before they would leave for the day and that they could march all day on that one cup of Kakao, which sounds a little bit fanciful, but isn't necessarily incorrect, because if you remember back to the old Max, I mentioned that the Cacao Bean is around 50 percent cocoa butter, which means there's a lot of calorie density in that hot chocolate.

So, it is quite possible that his army was marching all day on that. One of the other reputations that Cacao has that we assume is very modern also comes from Aztec times, and that's that Cacao or chocolate is an aphrodisiac. This is nothing new.

This is nothing that we've invented quite recently. This goes back to Aztec times, and it comes from Emperor Montezuma and the Spanish reporting that before he visited his harem of women; he'd be presented with a gold goblet filled with Cacao that he would consume beforehand.

In fact, the one of the Spaniards reporting on this said that he would consume 50 gold goblets of Cacao, but we could probably assume that he was exaggerating a little bit. The other thing that Cacao is used for in the Aztek times, which is fascinating, particularly the Spanish arrived; is it was the national currency.

So, these innocent little Cacao beans were, in fact, used as money. Mozza, Zuma himself had a warehouse full of millions and millions of Cacao beans. And whilst as an average layperson, you couldn't eat or consume Cacao, you would carry it on your person to buy things.

And if you look at the cost of living around that time, the Spanish arrived for, for example, one ripe tomato that would cost you one bean annually. Avocado would be three beans. A rabbit would cost you about 30 beans.

Or if you wanted to buy a sexual slave or human sacrifice, you'd be up for three thousand Cacao beans. The Spanish thought was fabulous because when they arrived in what is effectively Mexico now, that money grows on trees because cocoa beans grow on trees. In the meantime, they took all the gold, the silver and the copper out of the ground and took it back to Spain because it did take the Spanish a little while to cotton on how magical Cacao was. As much as they saw the Aztecs consuming it and revering it. It was still some time before it arrived in Spain.

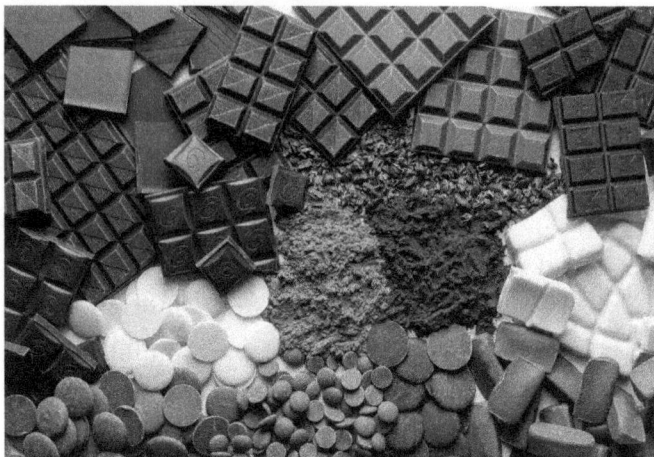

5. The history of chocolate - enter Europe

Now, you know about the Mesoamerican American history, which is really fascinating, particularly about how Cacao was really linked with those human sacrifices, but then we bring it to Europe, which I guess starts to shape it into something that we know and love today. So, we're still back in what is effectively Mexico, where the Spanish have arrived in the Aztec society and the first intersection of Europe.

And Kakao comes in 15 NITU, and it comes thanks to Christopher Columbus. Take yourself back to 15 NITU. And what we've got, we've got Christopher Columbus and his Spanish entourage who have just seized a canoe off the island of what we now know is going to harbor, which is of Honduras.

And within that canoe there's a number of locals and they hold out an offering of cocoa beans to the Spanish. Now we have, fortunately, some really long-lost records of what happened from Christopher Columbus, a son. But as these are being held up now, you have to imagine the Spanish had no idea what these were.

They look like dried up almonds to them. They held no value. But everything we've learned about the Aztecs, the Mayans, the mix, they revered them. They were precious to them. So you have Christopher Columbus take them and some of them are discarded on the bottom of the canoe.

And the reports are that the indigenous people, that the eyes were as big as saucers because they couldn't believe something so precious had been discarded. And the other note is that they stooped to pick them up as if someone had dropped an eye.

So this is really wonderful imagery about this first intersection of Cacao and European society. But it's always quite low for a while. That's in 15 two in the 15 20s, a shipment of Cacao does arrive in Spain on a ship full of all these marvelous things from the new world.

So you can imagine all the things arriving in the Spanish court, how well the king, Carlos, was a little bit preoccupied with various political things going on. And whilst we can assume a cup of Cacao had been made for him, it really didn't take off and it wasn't really seeing much in Spain. However, in the new world, in Central America and so forth, colonization was happening, and Cacao plantations were growing. And in fifteen, eighty-five, we find that Cortez brings back a shipment of Cacao to Spain. And this time it takes off. And the Spanish are intoxicated with this exotic, amazing, luxurious drink that comes from the new world.

However, cocoa beans are a short supply. They're very, very, very expensive. And it really remains the secret of the Spanish court for some time. It becomes very ritualized in the Spanish court. It's had for breakfast. It's had on special occasions that very much secret.

Where it starts to leak out to Europe is when Princess Anne from Spain marries into the French Quarter, marries I always forget the Louis Kings, but married one, I think Louis the 13th. And with that, she took Cacao with her, and she took her habitual cup of Cacao every morning for breakfast to the French court.

And the French don't hold back. They love it and they go crazy for it. And as soon as the French court cottons onto this, this is in the early sixteen hundreds, it spreads to the rest of France. And with that, it eventually makes its way to England.

And this is where we see a really big change in chocolate is thanks to the English, would you believe? But then again, maybe it's of no surprise, given that we have a lot of brands that exist still today, like fries and Cadbury's and so forth.

So it arrives in England. Now, remember, we're not talking about chocolate at this point. We're still talking about hot chocolate or a drink. And what you see popping up in England is chocolate houses. If you may have heard about tea houses and coffee houses like chocolate. These are all products coming in from the new world, all very glamorous, very exotic and very expensive.

And with that, we're seeing chocolate houses where aristocracy, well-to-do people would meet to indulge in some hot chocolate talk business and talk politics.

As the new world was expanding and this was all popping up in London, you had the cheapest of all of these houses was the coffee houses. This was followed by tea houses. Tea houses cost about twice that of coffee houses.

And then you had chocolate houses, which were about double that of the tea houses. And there's one particular chocolate house in London that I love the description, the contemporary descriptions of.

And it's probably the most famous from the late 60s and hundreds. And it was White Chocolate House and the temporary descriptions that it was the most decadent how on earth. And it was all fueled by this luxurious glob called chocolate. And this all this concept.

And it's a little bit how we view it in a way. Now, there's all this concept of this exotic thing is decadent and it's driving depravity and so forth that has wonderful imagery around it.

So the chocolate houses exist in London for a while. But the question is, how do we get from this drink to what we know now, which is a bar of chocolate and the fascinating journey that we go through because we're talking about the late 16 hundreds now and we're still drinking chocolate.

And it was still quite some time before we started to get a chocolate bar. And we can thank the English again for the first chocolate bar. And I wonder if you've heard of the brand Frys.

If you've been in England, you may know fries, orange cream or fries, peppermint cream, and in 1847 they worked out how to make a block of chocolate. So we have them to thank to begin with, not quite what we know now.

This block, which is an exceptional block from Covay's who are Australian makers here in Melbourne. If I eat this, this is going to be creamy. It's going to be smooth. It's going to be sweet. It's going to be all of these things that we associate with chocolate.

Amazing quality, of course, but that first bar in nineteen forty-seven that fries made was very different to this because the cocoa bean is actually quite gritty by nature. And it's not until the late eighteen hundreds that we start to see smooth chocolate as we start to see more industrialized processing of chocolate.

So, fries were just grinding up chocolate and mixing the, the pieces of chocolate with cocoa butter and gritty sugar. Sugar wasn't refined then. This was still quite new, still quite exotic coming from the new world and they would mold it into a slab of chocolate.

So it was very, very inelegant. But people loved it and they continue to make this in very small batches until the eighteen sixties where they got more commercial about it. Now, at this time, we're starting to see a lot of industrialization, which just helped the chocolate industry along significantly.

So in the late 70s, we saw from thanks to the Swiss that milk powder was added to chocolate for the first time. Some argue that was a good thing. Some argue that it ruined chocolate. I'll leave it to you to decide. We see the invention by Lindt of the machine.

The machine will talk about it later, but that's what gives a smooth chocolate. And in England, we started to see apothecary's selling chocolate.

And what's interesting about those apothecary's is that a lot of the brands that we still have today, surprise was an apothecary, as was Rowntree, which is still sold in the U.K.

And we start to see Cadbury come on the market as well. And at that point, at the end of the eighteen hundreds and the start of the nineteen hundreds, you had this magical time for chocolate, and that is the cost of cocoa beans and sugar came down, industrialization increased, and you had an explosion of products hitting the market to the point that in a decade you had several hundred different chocolate products hitting the market in England alone.

And from that, that's the basis of the chocolate industry that we know and love today. And it's shaped what we know and love today. What we want to get from the history is all those wonderful stories, but we want them now to move past that same Cadbury recipe that's been around for over 100 years.

And we want to start to identify what is the world's best chocolate, which we're going to go through some more steps in a moment.

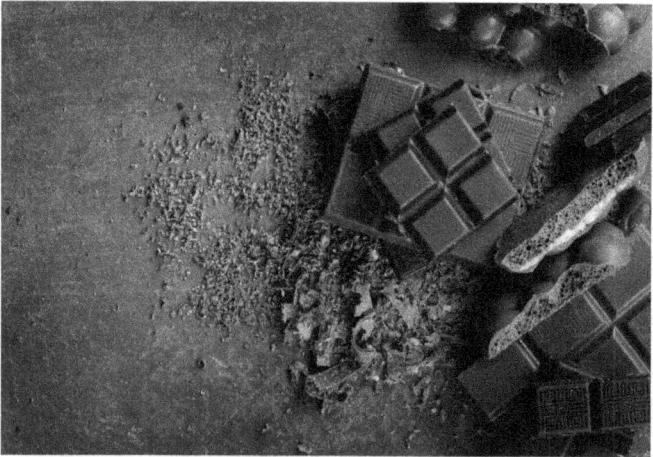

6. Single Origin vs Single Estate Chocolate

Another step that you can use to identify great chocolate is looking at whether it's marked as a single origin or single estate, and they're very important distinctions because when you go and pick up a block of chocolate and it says single origin, it sounds great. It sounds kind of fancy.

It sounds like it's going to be good. But is it? That's a really tough question to answer. I would suggest that when you see single origin, your approach with caution. So what single origin means is quite vague.

A lot of people think that it means like wine, that the grapes come from a particular vineyard. But it doesn't it means typically that it comes from a particular area. And if you pick up a single origin chocolate that comes from Peru, for example, that means that those beans come from Peru, which you're talking about, a land mass of, I think, one point three million square kilometers. So there's all that nuance that you get with a flavor bean.

So like grapes and like anything else that coffee beans, you're looking for microclimates for the concept of terra, which I can't pronounce. The French accent. And you're looking at how that microclimate influenced the flavor beans.

So when you're looking at a bean, a chocolate, it's made from beans from Peru. That could be all sorts of things thrown into the mix with non-complimentary flavor profiles and even different species.

One of the other problems we have, and this is if you don't have transparency about the bean, is specific beans and flavor profiles need to, for example, be roasted at different temperatures to bring out the flavor profile. Mass-market chocolate, for example, is bought on the market.

It's all put together, roasted at one temperature and you're getting a lot of tannins and bitterness and so forth in that. Just on a note about this, while we're talking about single origin and single estate. The other thing I'm going to throw into the mix for you is percentage is a guide only.

I was just talking to someone recently about this, and they commented on a sixty nine percent chocolate, that, oh, it doesn't taste bitter like I would expect a dark chocolate to taste. And that's because it was amazing quality beans.

When you've got cheap beans and or poorly processed beans, you're going to get bitterness in your chocolate. It's I can give you a sixty nine percent that tastes quite floral and light and put against a fifty five percent, for example, that actually has a very natural astringent, bitter taste.

And it's not about the percentage, it's about the quality of the beans. But we digress. We're going to get a single origin, bit of a misnomer, a bit of a vague term.

So if I pick up, for example, a packet of linked and single origin, I'm going to put two and two together and say Lynch is mass market chocolate. They're not going to have access to great beans, says single origin. But it's not going to mean much where it gets confusing.

And this is where you're going to have to use your chocolate detective skills is when you pick up a block of chocolate that says single origin. For example, we talked about Valrhona Manjiro obviously before. When you pick this up, this is single origin. It comes from Madagascar.

It has somewhere on the on the label that it's from Madagascar. So you can look at this and say, OK, Madagascar. Now, that's going to tell you a couple of things. First, we know that Madagascar is one of the top producing countries for quality beans in the world.

So with your little chocolate expert brain ticking away, you go to Madagascar. That's a chicken favorite this. But is this single origin good or not? And that's always hard to tell. But again, like with ethics, start to scratch the surface. For example, with Manjiro, if you look on Verona's website, what you'll see is that it comes from a particular valley in Madagascar, which I think is the San Marino Valley.

So whilst it's not a single estate or a single plantation coming from the one farm, it's in a really small pocket of land that's going to have the same microclimate. So that's going to tell me I'm going to take a chance on that chocolate.

That's probably going to be pretty good if it just said Madagascar and you couldn't find out any more information with that. I would probably to single origin. That's a very vague use of that term. It's not a well-regulated term.

Things, however, change when we talk about single estate or single plantation. And this is typically your chocolate detective brain should give this a big tick now or never guarantee your chocolate is great, but it's going to be a pretty good guess that it is.

So this one from Michelle Clouzot, for example, it'll be one of my favorite chocolates also comes from Madagascar. So on the label, you see Madagascar. But the difference is this is a single plantation.

The beans from this chocolate come from the same plantation year in, year out. And typically, the only people who are going to go to that much detail to care about going to the same plantation or the same estate every year to get that same type of profile are those chocolate makers who embrace art and science and produce beautiful chocolate. So what does that tell us? That tells us a number of things. Single plantation or single estate is generally a good chocolate. Single origin is a really vague term and approach it with caution and with that approach percentage with caution be open minded about percentage and use it as a guide only a little.

Another little tip about how to identify good chocolate. Good quality producers rarely have the percentage first and foremost on the packaging. It's normally quite discreet on the packaging.

This example, it's just quite small down the bottom. Some brands you even have to look on the back to find the percentage. What that tells us is that they are potentially looking to exploit a flavor profile in that bean. They're not just trying to sell you something on a percentage basis because percentage is a guide.

Only single estate or single plantation is great. A distinct a discrete use of percentage is potentially good, single origin could go either way.

7. A Sensory Experience - How to Taste

So we've talked a lot about chocolate and hopefully you're starting to think about what you can buy and the things that are going to tell you whether a chocolate is good or bad or amazing. And hopefully you're aiming at the amazing.

But of course, all this is pointless unless you know how to taste chocolate. So we're going to start to talk about taste and hopefully you've got some chocolate with you and you're going to taste along with me.

Now, a few things to learn about taste is a bit easy on yourself. The problem is there's a lot of purists in the tasting world, whether it's chocolate, whether it's whiskey, whether it's coffee, whether it's wine.

And I don't know about you, but I know that I used to pick up a bottle of wine and I'd read the label on the back, and it would be really difficult to relate to what they were trying to describe. And you'd have very poetic things just described, like it tastes like the first dew on the grass on a spring morning or something like that. So don't worry about all of that. We're going to give you some really simple tips on how you can start to identify flavor in chocolate and really start to heighten your experience and be that chocolate expert with that.

The other thing to remember about taste that I think this is really cool is it's highly individualized. So what I taste, what you taste, what your friend tastes, it's always going to be different. And there's a number of reasons for this.

But one of those reasons is the way that taste is one of our five senses, works and taste works differently from the rest of our senses because taste goes through the creative side of the brain instead of the logical side.

And with that, it starts to tap into all of your memories. And with that, of course, our memories are different, our experiences are different. But that's what's going to start to trigger your brain to identify taste.

So the beautiful thing is if I say something in your tasting, something completely different, that's fine. It's just the way that it's going to be. So your palate is your palate and its individual. The other thing about taste is we're not really tasting perse.

We're largely smelling, and we should be using all five of our senses. And we're going to talk about how to use all of those senses in just a moment to eat your chocolate. But taste is actually the act. Largely 90 percent of taste is the act of the aromas of the chocolate or whatever you're consuming actually going up the nasal cavity. And so that's why when you've got a cold, for example, and you're a bit blocked up in your nose and you lose your sense of taste, it's because your nose, your ability to smell influence is what you can taste. It's really good if you take something you don't like.

You can hold your nose and you mitigate a lot of that taste there. So let's get started with using your five senses, first of all. So I have a piece of chocolate here. So grab yourself a piece of chocolate.

Doesn't matter what it is at the moment, and we're going to start by site. We want to look at things first of all, now, of course, it isn't just about the chocolate. You can look at the packaging.

One of the great things that you have started to probably see through this masterclass is good quality. Chocolate often comes with beautiful packaging. So take a moment to enjoy it, look at it, touch it, feel it.

But when we're looking at our chocolate, what we've got with this particular piece is untampered piece of chocolate. So it's not quite so shiny, but you can look at the sheen or the lack of sheen and take that in on the back.

You want to have a look and see if there's any bubbles. It's an interesting thing about whether you see bubbles on your chocolate, because some would argue it's a sign of poor processing. But as with everything, there's a little bit of discretion with that, because if it's a small artisan producer, they may be producing by hand and that may lead to a few little bubbles.

That's fine if you're buying from a big company that's industrially processing. Bubbles are a bad thing. If your chocolate ever has that white bloom on it, you can still eat it. It's not going to do anything wrong to it means it's being exposed to heat and the CALBERT has risen to the top. I personally find that the texture changes and when the texture changes, the flavor changes.

But it's not going to make you sick. And then you want to look at the color. There's no right or wrong color for Cacao, but it does come in lots and lots of different colors, particularly in the dark chocolate. Is it a dark, rich brown? Is it a reddish brown? Is it a light brown?

It's just a nice point of distinction. Then we come to listening and you may be wondering, well, how do I hear chocolate? And that's easy because chocolate, one of the things we love about it is its distinctive snap.

So if I break this. That's what you want to hear, is that lovely snap, that snap is going to tell us two things. One is that there's a good amount of cocoa butter in that chocolate. And the second is that it is being well tempered or coarse.

This isn't tempered chocolate, but lots of cocoa butter. Don't assume your chocolate has cocoa butter. It's always good to read the labels because cocoa butter is used in the cosmetics industry, which is quite a good price on the market. And a lot of industrial brands will skim from the cow butter and remove that and add vegetable oils and things like that into it instead.

So always, always read the ingredients label if you see vegetable oils or something or palm oil, if that's not going to be good chocolate, then we come to smell. So we're just going to initially.

Smell it, and these smells delicious, and I can't wait to eat it, the best time to smell chocolate is this piece is quite small. So is on the break when you're releasing all those aromatics, because we're going to come to this in a moment.

Chocolate, as with anything else, isn't about taste per say. It's about aromatics. And for me in this one, I'm getting this really thick, wonderful chocolate smell and it's really priming all my senses for that moment when I get to eat it.

And then we come to feel you just wrap between your fingers. That will release the oils a little bit. And of course, in a moment we're going to eat that piece of chocolate you've got if you haven't already and you're going to feel it in your mouth, of course.

And this is one of the most magical parts of experiencing chocolate, but not just tasting chocolate. We're experiencing it. The feel that you're going to get in the mouth, feel that you're going to get when you eat your chocolate.

It's a very, very particular thing because the magic about cocoa butter is it's the only fat that is solid at room temperature that melts up 37 degrees.

And what else is 37 degrees or thereabouts? It's the human body. Your body is perfectly primed to melt chocolate, and how magical is that? And now we're about to come to taste.

So there's a lot to say about taste. First up is taste is a very, very limited term. So there's a thing called a tongue map and that tells us where we taste the five different flavors that exist in the world. Do you know what those are? I had to go and look them up to make sure it was definitely five.

There is sweet, there is salty, there is umami, there is sour and bitter, I think. Please feel free to correct me if I'm wrong with that. And each of those flavors are experienced at a different part of the tongue suite, for example, is the tip of the tongue umami, which is the new flavor, which is that sort of meaty, savory flavor is the midpoint of the tongue.

Bitterness is at the back of the tongue. And when we get to tasting what I find I do, I quite often point to different parts of my mouth where I'm experiencing things. And that's because your tongue has a flavor map. But flavors are different for aromas.

We have five flavors, but we have hundreds and hundreds and hundreds of aromas and this is what we're really tasting. But with that comes complexity, how do you identify one particular aroma over the hundreds that there are? And this is why we have the flavor wheel. And if you're doing this masterclass with the tasting, you'll have a copy of this flavor, Will. Otherwise, you'll have a link of where to find it on my website. And this is a great tool.

This helps to guide you through what you are tasting. National Geographic did a study a few years ago where they surveyed, I think it was several million people on taste. And the simplified version of what they found is that most people are terrible tasters.

Most of us don't know what we taste. We can identify very basic things. We identify flavors well; we know if we like things or not. If I ask you to identify a specific, that's very difficult for a lot of us. For the record, if you are a 16-year-old female, you are the best taster.

Women are better tasters and the older you get, apparently the worse you get. But we can train ourselves to be good tasters and we can use tools like the flavor wheel. And how this works is you've got the inside circle, which has really basic flavors to it.

So it has things like fruity or nuts, just really basic things, spicy. It's you don't have to overthink it. It is really, really valid to say it tastes fruity, for example. As your palate develops and you get better at identifying things, you move to the mid circle, and this is just where we get a little bit more specific. So instead of saying it's fruity, you might be able to identify that it tastes like citrus or taste like berries. Or instead of saying that it's spicy, you might be able to identify Brown Spice, for example. Finally, and I must admit, I don't think I'm here. You move to the outside circle, and this is where things get very, very specific.

Sometimes that's a little bit more obvious than others. For example, we've gone from pretty citrusy, you might now say, rather than citrusy, you might say lime or lemon, you may be able to distinguish between the two or grapefruit or instead of saying berries, you might be able to identify, identify raspberries as a flavor.

And some of those will come more naturally to you than others. And again, you just relax into it. There's no right or wrong. It's a process of learning. It's a process of fun and just enjoy it. With that, I will note down the bottom here, there's a wonderful set of descriptions which I like to point out, and these are valid flavors. I don't know if they're particularly pleasant flavors, but you have rubber, you have skunky, you have petroleum and you have medicinal or valid flavors.

Certainly, one of the chocolates I'll be showing you today has a very strong tobacco flavor. I'm not a smoker, but I like the tobacco flavor. So that's a lot of talking, not a lot of tasting yet. Are you ready to try some chocolate is my question. OK, you should have your piece of chocolate.

It doesn't need to be big. What I want you to do with it is pop it into your mouth, take a couple of small bites and use your tongue to move it around your mouth and just concentrate on that flavor now, don't you? A lot. If you chew, you release all those aromatics quite violently and you're not going to get the flavor profile. It's a gentle, considered experience. So just let it melt. You will find the flavor comes in waves.

So it will start with a particular flavor. There'll be a midpoint and an end point. And then you'll also want to focus on how it lingers. Now, it depends on what chocolate you're eating. If you are eating some of the world's best chocolate, you're going to have a great flavor profile.

If you're eating Cadbury or Hershey or Lynch, you may not be getting much, but that's okay. It is what it is. Let's go ahead and eat some chocolate. And I always struggle eating on camera. I feel very self-conscious. But I find it such a joy to eat good chocolate, so I'm eating Valrhona, Guano 70 percent and it starts off really smooth and then brings in this really masculine bitterness.

And for me now, it's easing off on this toasty coffee, a little bit acidic fruity flavor. And it's just changed his profile quite considerably. Very strong lingering in my mouth at the moment, I know this chocolate well, I know continues to linger strongly. And it's very much about that taking that journey.

8. It Starts with a Bean | Bean to Bar Processing

I hope you enjoyed tasting some chocolate and particularly that you had some marvelous chocolate to taste. We'll get to some more tasting shortly, including working through dark milk. And if you're tasting with my masterclass, the world's first ever blonde chocolate as well, which I love sharing with people.

But before we get to that point, it's really cooled to know how this little fella, the humble kalbi, becomes your favorite chocolate bar. The fascinating thing about the cow beans is they grow in these pods that we're aware of. We talked about them through the history.

We've talked a little bit about the colors that the Mayans, because of the reds and the vibrant purples, believed the gods had shed their blood on the cocoa beans. But they also come in vibrant yellows and vibrant oranges. But in those pods, you've got around 40 Cacao things. But the fascinating thing is, at this point in their raw state, they actually don't taste like anything which surprises most people. There's no chocolate flavor at this point.

I've been lucky enough to try some raw cocoa beans and I would describe them as a bland lychee. But what the campaign does have with these 40 beans in a pod is they're surrounded by all these thick, sweet white pulp.

And this is going to be really important in bringing out the flavor of chocolate in these beans. So got these really beautiful pods. We've got that 40 beans per pod with this white sweet pulp. The first step in processing is to harvest them from the trees.

Obviously, the pods are then cracked open, and those beans and all that pulp are scooped out to be fermented. And this is a really, really critical part of exceptional chocolate. So when I earlier said that chocolate is art and science mixed, this fermentation process requires both art and science because fermentation is the first stage of imparting flavor into those beans.

So that mixture is all scooped out ideally and in a traditional setting. It's laid out on banana leaves in the sun, and it's left there for several days in the heat and just turned every now and then to help the activation of that fermentation. And it's left there. And all that sweet white pulp becomes muesli and drains away. So it sounds really gross, but this is so critical. I can't stress enough how important this fermentation process is in giving you quality chocolate, get this fermentation process wrong. And even if you've got the best beans in the world, you're going to have really poor chocolate.

Now, there's some really cool products entering the market, and Valrhona is one of those with this particular chocolate that's actually double fermented, this chocolate is I I'm sure I'm pronouncing this incorrectly. It you could just it's a 55 percent Brazilian chocolate, but they double for mint.

So they go through that fermenting process to begin with as per normal to bring out the flavor of the chocolate. But then they add some local passionfruit pulp into the chocolate and that the sugars in the passion fruit pulp activates a second fermentation. And with that, that passion fruit flavor, they do it with banana as well.

That passion fruit flavor is naturally part of the chocolate. And when you eat it, you get this strong bit of Brazilian. Fifty five percent chocolate, but this really distinct acidic passionfruit flavor as well as it's not flavor added, it's through the fermentation process.

So beans are fermented, the next step is they need to be dried, and this is really interesting from a number of ways. Good quality produces the ones that grow. Cacao for the world's best producers is going to let those dry out in the sun quite naturally. And that's what you really want. What's happening with a lot of the Cacao out there that's not from these amazing brands that we've been talking about is a number of things. First is through economies of scale, they're trying to get through this drying process really quickly.

They put the beans into tents or huts with kerosene heaters to try and quicken that drying process. The problem you have with chocolate and with kickout, both a very, very porous.

So another little hinge is never stole your chocolate next to your blue cheese because it is going to absorb some of those smells. And of all the things that go together in the world, I don't think blue cheese and chocolate particularly do.

So if you can imagine Hutz full of cocoa beans drying with kerosene heaters, you going to have those cocoa beans take on some of that kerosene flavor. So this is another reason you don't want to be eating some of that cheaper chocolate.

It's going to have cheaper processing behind it. And I don't know about you. I don't want kerosene flavored chocolate. The other interesting reality about how chocolate is dried is you have a lot of small subsistence sized farmers who are producing cocoa and selling it on to co-ops.

They don't have great drying facilities. What they do is they spread the cocoa beans out along the roadside and dry them there, which is fine. But later, when we get to winnowing one of the parts of the process, this is where you start to find all sorts of interesting things in your cocoa beans, to be fair. This happens to the good companies as much as it happens to the poor quality, maybe a little bit more to the poor quality.

But all sorts of interesting things end up in your cocoa beans. For those who are buying a cow that's being dried on the side of the road, it's particularly bad because you get things like nuts and bolts, you get bullets, you get people who have found teeth in chocolate.

All sorts of weird and wonderful things end up with those cocoa beans. The good news, however, is they do get removed as part of the processing. So we go through fermentation, we go through dry. Now, hopefully drawings being done properly. It's really fascinating what the mass market brands will buy with their cocoa beans when it comes to quality.

Obviously with cow means, as with anything else you're drawing, they're drawing these cocoa beans in order to put them into huge sacks of cocoa beans and shipped them to the other side of the world aware of there being processed.

Now, if they haven't been dried properly, that's going to be a bit of a nasty mess. You're going to get mold. You're going to get all sorts of disgusting things going on there. And there is recognition in from some of the better producers in the industry quite publicly that mass market brands don't necessarily care all the time. If they get some moldy or infested beans, they will still process them anyway.

Another reason you don't want to eat mass-market chocolate, so they're dried the shift. Now, all of this happens in the growing country and something that's important to note. And if you think about that band of countries, we saw earlier that produce Cacao Cocoa is grown in developing countries and typically shipped to first world countries for processing. That means that the poorest people in this supply chain are in the growing countries.

The richest are in the first world. Countries that act of growing, harvesting, fermenting, drawing and distributing is all done in the growing countries. Typically, then we come to the first world countries, whether it's Switzerland, France, Australia, wherever it might be.

And the next step in processing is really important to the flavor profile, as important as fermenting, and that is roasting. And it's one of the reasons why with raw chocolate and for people who don't like to eat cooked foods, you're never going to get the same flavor profile from abroad chocolate because it isn't roasted roasting helps to bring out the flavor profile of chocolate, plain and simple.

As we mentioned earlier, depending on the chocolate where it's come from, that microclimate, that that flavor profile, that microclimate contributes to each different thing, not individually, but from a plantation, is going to require a different roasting temperature.

Mass-market chocolate pops it all in its roasted together, its astringent. It's bitter, it's volatile and its flavor, beautiful chocolate. We know what the art artisan chocolate maker knows, what the roasting profile is, and they rose to that particular one to bring that flavor out.

If you're not doing that, that's like a winemaker treating all grapes the same when they're making wine. It's probably not going to end so well. It's a good quality. Ones were raised very specifically.

We then move on to winnowing, which is where the bean is crushed and we're starting to extract the accounting and the actual Cacao that we're going to use for the chocolate. This is also through agitation. Normally in a factory, this is where all those oddities end up in your chocolate are removed.

And it's a pretty good process that you're only getting the Cacao from this point, from winnowing. We then go to conchie and crunching is a really cool process. And I will give credit to linked to this because they did invent the conch machine.

And to be fair to Lynch, whilst it is supermarket chocolate, what they do really well is they create really smooth chocolate because as we alluded to earlier, chocolate by nature isn't smooth. They say a particular brand in Italy, you'll find similar things in Mexico, this brand, but they don't want their chocolates, then it's smooth it out.

So, this chocolate is still Graney has almost a Sanit texture and delivers flavor in a really different way. But from the eighteen hundreds, we've gotten used to having the conch machine to make smooth chocolate. And that's what we associate with good quality chocolate. So conch is heated. Roller's the Cacao, though the chocolate runs through this for hours and hours and hours to make smooth chocolate, and it also releases volatile aromatics and therefore improving the flavor of your chocolate.

So really important to getting that flavor profile right as well. Good quality companies can Kunz for up to 72 hours over three days the likes of Cadbury. Maybe they there for a few hours. So again, there's always going to be a little bit of a difference with that. We're nearly at the end of the chocolate production cycle.

We then have chocolate in our little pieces, whether it's in little drops or circles or any of those shapes. And from this point, you have chocolate that's pretty tempered. And then the next step is to temper it or pre crystallization.

And that's the process of heating chocolate to a particular temperature, cooling it down to a particular temperature. And through that and the chemical structure of the chocolate, you stabilize the crystals in the chocolate. And from our perspective, as people who love to eat chocolate, it does two things. Temperature or pre crystallization is the other term for it. It makes chocolate really smooth.

And shiny and glossy, and it also helps to have that wonderful, distinctive snap that we associate with chocolate. Remember, that SNAP will also come from cocoa butter, but it will also come from good tempering. From that point, we can mold chocolate into whatever it is you're going to eat it as. So that's the process that we go through to make chocolate. I'm going to add one little other thing in here for you so that when you put your chocolate detective hat on, it's going to help you identify what's good quality chocolate. And actually, there's two things that are going to help you identify what's amazing quality.

There are two things to look for. First is, is your chocolate bean to bar Sabean to bar is a really cool term that's generally not always, but generally going to tell you a chocolate is good quality. And what it means, it means that chocolate here has controlled the whole supply chain from those cocoa beans, grown cocoa beans being grown through to being harvested, fermented, etc., all the way through to roasting and crunching and finalizing it as a product.

They've gone to source those beans for a particular flavor profile and really kept tight control of that all the way through. Bean to bar is cool. It means your chocolate maker is obsessive and artistic and creative and they're sourcing something very specific. Most chocolate chips aren't being. Most of them are what are called molders in the industry, and they buy buying their chocolate.

They look in a catalog, they see the chocolate they want, and they buy it in. They melted down and they make the block of chocolate they want or maybe they add a little bit of flavor, make individual chocolates.

Now, there's nothing inherently wrong with that. That's that is a big and legitimate part of the industry. But what I would be doing is I would be asking those chocolate chips a little bit about their chocolate. Now, if they're going to tell you that they have been to bioprocess, awesome, I would take that as a sign that they're probably making good quality chocolate.

If they tell you what my experience is, most tell you is if they tell you are we use a professional Belgian chocolate or a professional Belgian coverture, which is a name for a professional chocolate, if they're saying things like that, I would be approaching with caution, because if we go back to where does this chocolate come from, we know it doesn't come from Belgium.

Most chocolate is use it. Belgian chocolate has been really well marketed. And as consumers, we think it's the best. And most people would go, oh, that's great. But you're going to come out of this as a chocolate expert, so you already know better.

You're going to know that what they're doing when they say that is they're buying chocolate out of the catalog, not probably the best quality and then melting it down to make their product.

So I'd be a little bit more suspicious of that. Now, if they said we buy our chocolate from this really cool company in Ecuador or we buy our chocolate from this French company, for example, I would be more interested in what they're making. But I'd be really wary of the chocolate here who's not been Tabaha and hasn't controlled all that processing we've just talked about or who's being very generic and just using a Belgian chocolate because that processing matters. And again, it's about transparency. And you want a chocolate here. Who can tell you about the processing so you can understand if you're going to be eating a great chocolate or probably paying a lot of money for an ordinary chocolate.

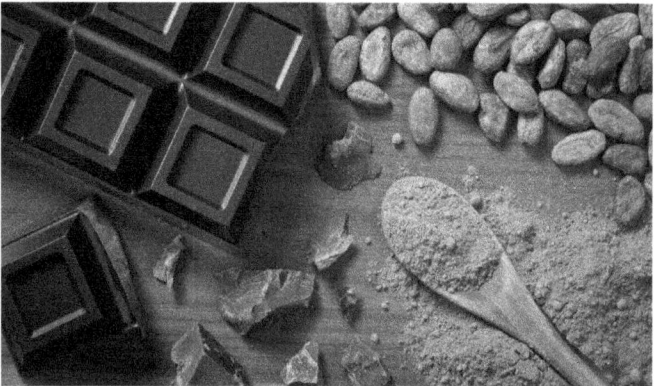

9. Taste with Me | Dark Chocolate

I've got some great news for you. We're about to eat some hot chocolate, which is really exciting. So what you need to have with you is obviously some chocolate with you. We're going to start with dark, really important thing.

And when you're tasting chocolate is to always start with dark before milk or white or anything. And that's because if you have a light, a chocolate, a milk chocolate to start with, the sugar in that chocolate is going to kill your palate.

And by the time you get to dark chocolate, you're not going to taste anything. It's just going to taste very bitter. So we're always going to start with that. If you're doing the tasting as part of my masterclass as well.

What you also can have with it is if you grab your flavor, will, that's a really useful tool and also grab your tasting notes, because that's going to have the details of what's included in your chocolate pack. I'll also include with this the chocolates that we're tasting. So if you're not getting the chocolate through the master class, you can hopefully go and find some of this yourself. And this isn't for everybody.

But I'm going to start really, really hardcore because I like it and we're going to start with 100 percent chocolate. So when I say it's not dark, it doesn't get much darker or doesn't get any darker than one hundred percent.

So the chocolate I'm going to be tasting is from Dumarce. It's actually probably my favorite brand in the world, this exceptional Italian brand from just outside of Turin who make beautiful, beautiful chocolate.

And this 100 percent is made entirely with that Cerillo Bean, which means that, as we discussed before, it's not going to have the same level of bitterness as some of the other beans. I will warn you, though, if you're milk chocolate lover and you start dabbling in one hundred percent, even if it's Dumarce or something of equal quality, it's probably going to knock your socks off.

I had someone taste some recently, not necessarily dark chocolate lovers, but they appreciated the experience. And this is how we want to approach all of your chocolate eating, approach it with a bit of playfulness and openness and just see where it takes you.

So 100 percent remember to use your five senses and listen, smile, look at it, feel, etc. Hopefully you've got some chocolate there now popping in your mouth, remember, don't you? Too much. Just a couple of small bites and work it through your mouth and see what you come up with. I'm going to taste this one and tell you a little bit about one hundred percent chocolate if you bear with me chewing on camera.

So it's really interesting as one hundred percent, it's not coming in with that huge slap of bitterness, it's really mild to start with. Very, very clean on the palate. And yes, there's a level of strong Cacao flavor, but there's a flavor profile of red berries and sweetness that's underpinning that.

And what I find with these really, really. Dark chocolate is a 99 percent, 100 percent is. They really cut your mouth very thick. I find it quite a luscious mouthfeel, I always describe it. It's like having mud cake in your mouth or something like that, which is just delicious to me.

Thick, luxurious, very Kakao, red berries, touches of honey. And for me, that's marvelous. What's interesting about this particular one from Dumarce is the quality of bean is amazing. So it comes in tiny packaging.

Twenty-five grams. But you need a tiny bit. I mean, I eat about the equivalent of that and got this rich, intense Cacao chocolate experience from it.

So a little goes a long way when you're dealing with one hundred percent. The other thing I should have mentioned that you will need with you when you're tasting chocolate is a glass of water or some other form of palate cleanser. It might not sound like a lot tasting a few chocolates, but it really does help to clear your palate, things that are useful water, probably particularly fizzy water, a particularly good dry biscuit, white bread, green apples, cucumber sorbet.

If you're really fancy, they'll all work really well. So next, we're going to move on to a 70 percent chocolate, and I love this chocolate. It's going to far from Valrhona. And here's my question for you. How does it sound familiar to all?

Because if you go back to when we were talking about Christopher Columbus arriving in Central America and seizing that that canoe, he did so off the island, Guam. So Valrhona has intentionally named its chocolate after that.

And what's really cool about this chocolate Valrhona, which is a boutique French brand, are always pushing the boundaries with chocolate and innovating. And they spent seven years researching this chocolate to take you back in time through eating it back to that moment in 15 02 when Christopher Columbus arrived in Honduras and what that Cacao at that time would have tasted like.

And with that, they've blended Cacao from lots of different regions and a blend is OK. I know we talked about single estate and single plantation are masterful. Blend is a masterful thing. And they've blended lots of different bean types from lots of different places to recreate that flavor.

Guam is also potentially the world's most iconic and well-known chocolate. When it was released in nineteen eighty-six, it was the world's first ever 70 percent chocolate, which just blew everybody's mind. And it was considered so bitter at the time that Valrhona sold it in little squares because people couldn't handle this bitterness. But it still really loved by pastry chefs and chefs all over the world.

And if you're fine dining and look at the dessert menu, you'll more often than not find chocolate desserts are made out of our own Iguanodon. So Guano has a 70 percent chocolate. So, it's a really nice point for people who like dark chocolate, those dabbling in it a little bit.

This is in the pre tempered pieces, which is why it looks not so shiny and so forth. I describe this chocolate as the GQ magazine of chocolate. So if you know GQ, it's all about men's fashion and lifestyle and it's masculine, but very elegant and very refined.

And this is what this chocolate is. So hopefully you've got some Valrhona going to hang with you. If not, grab some chocolate, particularly if you've got a 70 percent or something around that. And I'm just going to tell you what this tastes like and see what you think of yours.

So got that nice snap again. It's so different from the hundred percent that I've just eaten. It comes through is very nutty for me to begin with. Lots of roasted flavors. These powerful hitter Cacho starts to come through, which is we know that one house that has this elegant expansion of bitterness, bitterness is a flavor not as an unpleasant thing. And then you get coffee, fruits, acidic fruits. That's hosting us again, and we did dabble in a little bit of gunfire earlier in the session, and the thing that I know from this, I'm not going to make you sit here for minutes for me to describe this.

But in several minutes, I'll still be able to taste this in my mouth. Valrhona does a marvelous job at having long lingering chocolates, and Guanabara exemplifies that. And it's a really nice little point.

With your chocolate eating, you start rush the next piece, because when you're eating the world's best chocolate, it is going to linger, and you want to enjoy that moment sitting in your mouth. What did you think of the one you had? Now, great little tip, there's a thing in tasting called parallel tasting.

And you can take two products, it's not much she's showing you that, to be fair. Let's show you the blocks. You can take two products that are much the same percentage in this case and experience how different they are together, because, as we discussed before, percentages a guide only.

And with this, we've got the Valrhona going to higher, which is 70 percent. And I'm Michele Occlusal single plantation, which is from Colombia, which is sixty nine percent. So traditional chocolate buying would tell us they're much the same chocolate.

But if you can get hold of two chocolates that are the same or very similar percentages, you're going to find that they're completely different experiences. So after the Valrhona, I'm curious, try the Michelle Clouzot. Michelle Kazak is another French brand. They have a tagline of the noble ingredient and also known as the goldsmith of chocolate, and have been really particular about the minimal number of ingredients in their chocolate.

All of the good chocolate will have minimal ingredients. But for example, Michelle Kunze don't use soy lecithin, which I'm sure I always pronounce incorrectly, which is the emulsifier that a lot of chocolates use.

It's not necessarily an issue, but they just choose to leave it out because they're about the noble ingredients. So this particular plantation chocolate is going sixty nine percent, which I have a piece of here. Is much larger.

As soon as I. And really strong notes of honey coming through that for me, a little bit of licorice. I don't think I saw that on the notes, but I'm getting licorice with that. And very menthol. Oh, it's really interesting.

And now lots of biscuit flavors. Fascinating. I've only just discovered this chocolate myself, so this experience is really new to me. Definitely Bacardi towards the end, definitely lots of mint horn, really, really interesting chocolate.

I love that. And this is what we were talking about, this beautiful evolution of taste that a good chocolate is going to go through and it's just taking the time and literally I'm rushing it a little bit to talk to you but taking the time to just to let it unfold and let those flavors change as far as determining what those flavors are, usual flavor and also just don't stress about it. Just let whatever comes to your mind be what it is your brain will get in tune with. Your experiences are different to mine. You're going to taste what works for you.

One last chocolate before we move on to the milk ones. And don't forget, if you're tasting with me, just to have a little drink water or something in between, because I love to talk about this brand, which is República Dalia cow. Now in Australia. I can't get this in bathroom. I can only get it in pieces, but that's fine pieces.

Whilst they're not tempered, an amazing way to eat great quality chocolate at an even more affordable price, not the chocolate that expensive for the quality that it is, but it becomes even cheaper in this format. It's not shiny, it's not glossy, but it has the same flavor.

What I love about República Dalia cow is out of all the chocolate that I deal in, that is all really, really ethical. República del Cow is probably the most ethical because the Cacao is grown in in Ecuador.

In this case, this is a fifty six percent Ecuadorian chocolate, and they source all the milk, the sugar except from Ecuador or neighboring Peru or Colombia. But importantly, the chocolate is produced in Ecuador.

We've touched on a few times that cocoa is grown in developing countries quite often, particularly in Ghana and the Ivory Coast, with some really problematic issues around poverty and so forth. But then it's shipped to first world countries for processing. And it's those, first of all, countries that keep the profit. Respublika Jilka, how do the processing in Ecuador and I do that as a social enterprise to keep that money in the community and supporting the communities.

So if you're talking guilt free chocolate, this is probably is guilt free as it gets as with the others. You've got a lovely snap on it. This is a really different chocolate; this is made from the National Bee.

So when we talked about beans, this is the one that was almost extinct. It's three percent of the world's production and it has the national bee has a really distinct, robust, powerful chocolate flavor.

And even though it's fifty-five per cent, which is quite low for dark chocolate, it is very powerful. And it also has lots of floral notes when I'm smelling it, which is interesting. So let's see what happens if you're eating República Dalia Ecuador. Fifty six percent.

Again, completely so, so fascinating, despite the fact I spent my life eating chocolate. It always amazes me how different flavor profile, good quality chocolate has. This is incredibly smooth, very powerful.

Cacho from the stop. That what that Forelle turns into very white floral flavors. And it's now changing to become incredibly toasty. Very natty, very really overriding flavors of toast now. It's delicious. And as we said, it's guilt free. So how are you going with your chocolate? I hope you found something that you love in your dark chocolate. We're about to move on to milk chocolate. I would suggest having a little bit of a break before you move on to the milk chocolate just to give you a palate, time to adjust. Maybe write down some notes of what you really enjoyed about those dark chocolate, because you forget in the moment you remember. But as we move on, you do forget. And let's see if we can find you some great experiences. Milk, chocolate.

10. Taste with Me | Milk Chocolate

OK, so I hope you're ready to try some milk chocolate, particularly for your milk chocolate people who have been hanging out for this, I'm going to suggest for the most part that you do the same things we did with the dark.

And let's start with the darkest chocolate and work your way forward. But I'm going to take a little exception to that because I want to talk about this. You may recognize the purple color that this comes in.

And this is what most of us identify as chocolate is Cadbury. It's what we had as a kid. We eat it when I run my events in person. I give people a piece of Cadbury. Let's get that out of the way. And they have it before the good chocolate.

And I ask them, what do they think about it? And they got yeah, it's great. It's yummy, blah, blah, blah. Now maybe you have some of this in the house or maybe you're doing the masterclass with the chocolate edition, in which case you'll have a little bit of Cadbury. So I want to start out on the Cadbury first and see how this tastes. So I want you to pop that in your mouth, do what we did with the other ones and let me know what you think.

Because what's really interesting is people come in thinking this is what they like, and this is what they eat on a day-to-day basis. But your perception potentially changes very much. I'm not going to pop it in my mouth.

I know what happens when I have this. And we're going to return to Cadbury at the very end and see what happens if you don't have Cadbury in the house and you haven't got chocolate as part of the masterclass, grab some lint if you've got any other chocolate in the house, particularly if it's milk, and just see how it sits with the others.

It's a really interesting experience because milk, chocolate, a controversial thing. Now the chocolate purists will tell you it's all about dark chocolate because with dark chocolate, you're going to have that flavor profile really come out and be at its best. Once you start adding milk, as with adding milk to coffee, for example, you start to meet those flavors. But it doesn't mean it's a bad thing. It's just a different thing. I'm a dark chocolate lover.

I love all that flavor profile. But there's a particular chocolate I'm going to talk you through in a moment from Republican Dalia that I describe as crack cocaine. I can't get enough of this if I start eating it. So there is no right or wrong. One of the best things when people do chocolate tastings, and particularly when you've opened your mind and you've become this chocolate expert, one of the things that's really cool is to drop all these beliefs that we have, these limiting beliefs that people come in and say, oh, I don't eat dark chocolate, or they say I only eat chocolate if 70 percent or above.

And I think this comes from people who have been eating chocolate, this and Julie Bishop, for example, or they've been hooked into the sweetness. When I was a Cadbury acholic that I mentioned at the very start of this, I was hooked into the sweetness. I put my hand up to that.

So let's see what happens with milk, chocolate. So we're going to start dorkiest. And for me today, that means this particular chocolate here, which is a marvelous brand here in Australia, that they make it locally. They hand grind all the cocoa and do the small batch artisan production they named Cuvee.

This particular chocolate is Saleel. It's forty two percent. The beans come from the Solomon Islands. Amazing social enterprise behind this fascinating chocolate. I love getting people to try this. Number one, I personally believe that most good chocolate is forty percent and above.

Now, there are some exceptions to that, but you really need to be getting that 40 percent cocoa solids to get a quality milk chocolate. As a comparative point. Cadbury dairy milk in Australia is twenty six percent cocoa solids. That's the legal minimum requirement in Australia for chocolate to be called chocolate. Anything below that, it's called chocolate confectionary or compound chocolate. Interestingly, I did some research on this just yesterday because

I was curious what the Cacao content is in in the United States for it to be chocolate. And it's just ten percent for it to be called chocolate, which is quite remarkable. But what we're talking about is forty three percent here now, milk, chocolate. So it's going to be more muted, but it's still going to have a flavor profile because of those great beans if this one's quite thick.

So my snap requires a bit of extra effort. Now, this is a really interesting chocolate because when I smell this one and I know what it tastes like, but it smells really smoky and because I know what it tastes like, I'd go as far as tobacco, it smells in a pleasant way. A little bit like sitting by a campfire. The beautiful light brown color.

I just want to have a smaller piece in my mouth, excuse all the breaking. Let's see what it tastes like. Definitely, sweetness starts with compared to the darker chocolates. Let's smokiness comes in to begin with really smoking tobacco. But it's fascinating because it's really blended with these caramel chains, with this milk chocolate and very.

Milky, nutty, caramel, smoky Chines, which sounds like the most peculiar combination. Little bits of honey a little bit sweeter at the end. But a delicious, smooth caramelized milk chocolate with a really unique smokiness to it, just so you know, that smokiness comes from two things. It comes from, first of all, the bean. These particular beans from the Solomon Islands are grown and really volcanic soil.

Again, it's this concept of terra. The growing conditions are going to contribute to the flavor. And secondly, it's that Khiva, as an artisan producer, use unrefined cocoa butter, whereas a lot of small batch producers are using refined cocoa butter and by nature, that has a different flavor profile to it.

So how is your milk chocolate for the first one? Hopefully you're enjoying milk as much as the dog. OK, so let's move on. I'm going to talk about the Republic, Adel Cacho, 40 percent. This is the one I call crack cocaine. This is the same day, the same Nacio male being from Ecuador as the 56 percent that I talk to you threw in the dark chocolate.

And it still has that robustness. And this is the beautiful thing. When you have a high Cacho percentage in your milk, chocolate is still going to get a touch of bitterness and a touch of robustness through. But this is very cool because aside from all the ethical elements this comes with, this is also caramelized this chocolate.

And it actually has that on the packaging. And what they do is they use quite an ancient technique to add milk to the chocolate and they caramelize the milk, so they gently heat the milk before it goes into the chocolate, and it gives it a very distinct caramel flavor. Let's get tasting quite good again. I like this so much. It really does have a gentle hit of Cacho. It's. For me, I have to explain how I feel about this. This takes everything that you love about milk, chocolate, everything is a kid you loved about milk, chocolate, and it wraps you up in that coziness and warmth, but just in a more elegant adult way. Look, as a complexity.

As far as complexity goes, it's not here as with milk chocolates, generally, you don't get that level of complexity. What you're doing is getting a really gentle sweetness. You're getting a distinct caramel tone through that. You're getting elements and nuttiness, a little bit of a tiny, tiny touch of bitterness with that. Just a really nicely balanced milk chocolate that's far beyond your Cadbury or your lunch. That's going to give you a very different experience. Only problem with this chocolate is it does come in pieces, and you eat it by the handful, which is the worst thing I can say about this.

Chocolate is really delicious. So how did you go with your chocolate with that one, because we're about to move on to not only unique chocolate, but it's also by far my best-selling chocolate. So if you're tasting along with the chocolate as part of the master class, we're moving on to Valrhona Dulcie. If not Valrhona, which is the French brand, is probably one of the more accessible chocolate brands that you can get out there, and this is the world's first blonde chocolate, and I would argue the best example of one chocolate out there. So what is one chocolate is the question. And blonde chocolate is an accident. So blonde chocolate is caramelized. And it was an accident at Valrhona that a pastry chef left some white chocolate, 32 percent white chocolate in a bakery overnight or for a few hours longer than intended, came back and that white chocolate had caramelized having brought in all these toasted shortbread flavors.

And they tasted it. And it's like, wow, this is amazing. These tastes phenomenal. We need to make this. However, it wasn't so easy to make it at a commercial level. It took them six or seven years of research. Again, Valrhona are always researching and innovating before they had something they could release to the market pastry chef.

The pastry chef loved this because they used to be up righted Valrhona deuces putting white chocolate in the oven to try and bake it to get this gold and caramelized chocolate. But what if a pastry chefs think? I think it all comes down to the consumer and consumers love it. And as I said, it's by far my best seller.

What's phenomenal about it is all those people who come and say, no, I only like dark chocolate, I don't like milk chocolate. So many of them are fans of this and end up buying it. So let's give this a go.

By the way, as a note, there's some other brands, mass market brands that have started making what looks like a bland chocolate lately, wolves in sheep's clothing. I would describe it as its and if you look at the back, it will be flavor added to this. This is not flavor added to this chocolate. This is the process of that heating of the sugars that causes caramelization. So let's give it a go. So as soon as you smell it, you get caramel tones to sweet caramel tones.

And it is very delicious. It's such a unique chocolate, so it's sweet, but it's not overly sweet. It is full it starts off a little bit like creme Brule, which I love and really moves onto this distinct buttery shortbread.

The tones and what's fascinating about it is right at the very end, you get this hint of salt that kicks into it, which of course isn't so added to the chocolate. It's just the flavor. And any time we're talking about these flavors, inherent and flavors that are in your tasting notes, these are not flavors added to the chocolate.

These are flavors that are part of that flavor. Bean. And this is why this chocolate is amazing, because they are having these exceptional flavor things influence what you're experiencing. It's really delicious, quite clean on the palate, it doesn't linger like the dark chocolates linger way to moreish, potentially. I'm going to give you a little insider a tip, though.

I think I've still got some chocolate here. Our Valrhona Dulce, along with Valrhona Guano heart together, sandwiched together, pop them in your mouth at the same time. My little insider tips. That is an amazing combination. Highly, highly recommend you do that. And it does speak to the playfulness, which I think it's great to approach chocolate because you only find out such great combinations by trying them. My other little tip is going to be particularly with dark chocolate, but you could do the same with milk if that's your preference. If you like nuts in your chocolate, for example, I'm not a big fan of buying chocolate with nuts in it.

I find often the nuts are not of great quality and they're a little bit stale and the experience isn't that great. But go and get yourself some dry roasted almonds, for example, good quality, dry roasted almonds, pop them with a dark chocolate in your mouth. At the same time, you'll never look back.

You'll never buy chocolate with nuts in it again. So there's an elephant in the room. But there's one last thing that we need to talk about. And I'm actually passionate about this. And it's this thing. So he's a question is white chocolate? What do you think? Because I know what I get told by people all the time and they come along to events, and I'm often told white chocolate isn't chocolate at all.

And I question where that comes from. And it's this whole mythology about things we understand about chocolate. White chocolate isn't chocolate. The best chocolate comes from Belgium, etc.

And here's why. This particular chocolate from Michelle Occlusal, which is elegize it's thirty-three-point five percent cowslips, so it's got a lot of cocoa in it. So it's got significantly more canal Cacho than the Cadbury. Twenty six percent. Plus, Michelle Occlusal are using great quality beans. Cadbury are using cheap and nasty means of potentially dubious ethical qualities. So I would question what chocolate this has occurred so it doesn't have to count Massenet, it has cocoa butter, it's thirty-three-point five percent cocoa butter, but it comes from the raw ingredient, I would argue, with a better-quality bean and more of the raw ingredient that want a good quality white chocolate. It deserves the title a chocolate more than Cadbury does.

And let's try a little bit of this, because the other thing. Sounds obvious but smells like really the other thing that's interesting about white chocolate is a good quality white chocolate with that high Cacao percentage doesn't taste really sweet. Part of the problem is we've been eating cheap white chocolate that's full of sugar.

And as a result, we think it's an overly sweet. Not much else product, but with this one. So, Cranney, to stop. Less sugar than Cadbury because it's got more of the cow in a. And it tastes like panna cotta is this beautiful, unctuous, delicious. The moment the taste like Penikett is remembering also cow about a mouse at 37 degrees.

So when you've got a lot of cow, about a thirty three point five percent, which now I'm sure I've said many times, you get the mouthfeel is delicious and it's not overly sweet at all. It's just gentle, unfolding, creamy panna cotta deliciousness. So give white chocolate a go if it's good quality.

And avoid the cheap white chocolate. Which brings us back to our friend Cadbury. So if you've got a piece of again, if you're tasting along this part of the masterclass in your chocolates being provided, you should have a second piece of Cadbury. If you've just got some chocolate at home, otherwise grab that or come back to this at another time or have an experiment and have a taste of Cadbury.

I'm going to do it for you. I'm going to have a taste and sacrifice my taste buds to see what happens. And I'm going to be very open minded and have a genuine response. But this is the difference of amazing chocolate versus mass market. Biting at let's so soft. What's.

Everything about that is so different. The texture. Is odd, where is the good quality chocolate was really mounting beautifully and unfolding in your mouth. This is just oily and clings to your palate. And it just tastes enormously of sweetness. There's no Cacho flavor, there's no chocolate flavor because it's not made from a flavor bean.

It's made from mass market. Nasty things. Remember the forestry bean? It's like the supermarket tomato tastes like nothing. That's what that is. It tastes like nothing. If you just want to hit a sweetness, you can just go and have a teaspoon of sugar because that's what that tastes like.

No offense to Cadbury, of course, but vast, vast difference between good quality chocolate and your mass-market chocolate. And for me, I know which one I prefer. How's a tasting of milk chocolate gone? I hope you've been converted to the slightly darker chocolate.

11. Secret ingredient which makes chocolate taste so good

Whether baked as chips into a cookie, melted into a sweet warm drink or molded into the shape of a smiling bunny, chocolate is one of the world's most universally consumed foods.

Even the biggest chocolate lovers, though, might not recognize what this ancient food has in common with kimchi and kombucha: its flavors are due to fermentation. That familiar chocolate taste is thanks to tiny microorganisms that help transform chocolate's raw ingredients into the much-beloved rich, complex final product.

In labs from Peru to Belgium to Ivory Coast, self-proclaimed chocolate scientists like me are working to understand just how fermentation changes chocolate's flavor. Sometimes we create artificial fermentations in the lab. Other times we take cacao bean samples from real fermentations "in the wild." Often, we make our experimental batches into chocolate and ask a few lucky volunteers to taste it and tell us what flavors they detect.

After decades of running tests like this, researchers have solved many of the mysteries that govern cacao fermentation, including which microorganisms participate and how this step governs chocolate flavor and quality.

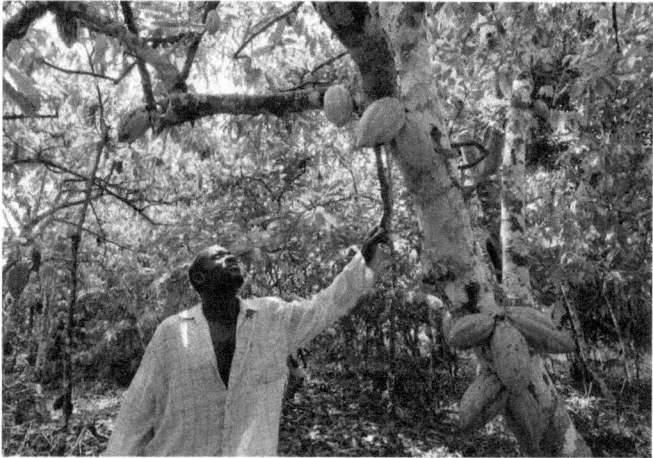

A plantation owner in Ivory Coast checks the pods on one of his cacao trees.

From seed pod to chocolate bar

The food you know as chocolate starts its life as the seeds of football-shaped pods of fruit growing directly from the trunk of the *Theobroma cacao* tree. It looks like something Dr. Seuss would have designed. But as long as 3,900 years ago the Olmecs of Central America had figured out a multi-step process to transform these giant seed pods into an edible treat.

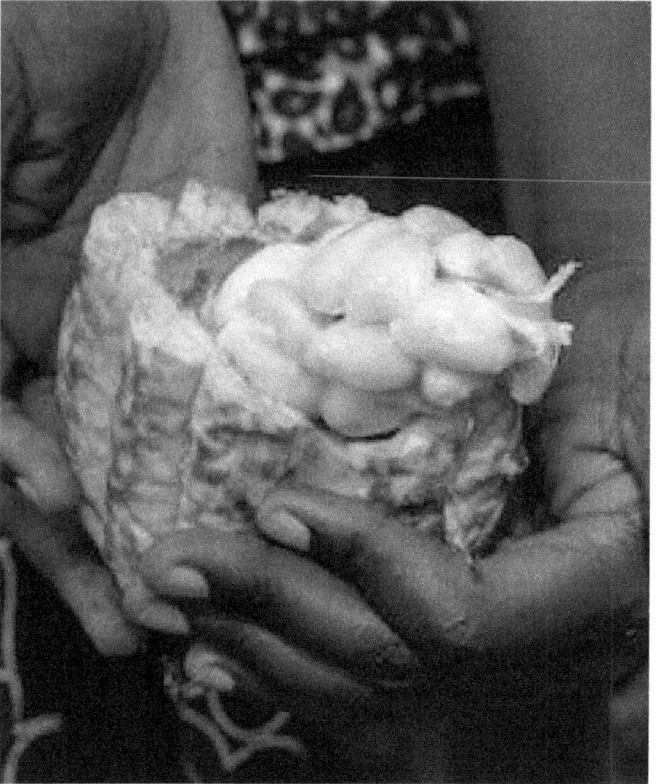

Inside the pods are seeds and pulp

First, workers crack the brightly colored fruit open and scoop out the seeds and pulp. The seeds, now called "beans," cure and drain over the course of three to 10 days before drying under the Sun. The dry beans are roasted, then crushed with sugar and sometimes dried milk until the mixture feels so smooth you can't distinguish the particles on your tongue. At this point, the chocolate is ready to be fashioned into bars, chips or confections.

It's during the curing stage that fermentation naturally occurs. Chocolate's complex flavor consists of hundreds of individual compounds, many of which are generated during fermentation. Fermentation is the process of improving the qualities of a food through the controlled activity of microbes, and it allows the bitter, otherwise tasteless cacao seeds to develop the rich flavors associated with chocolate.

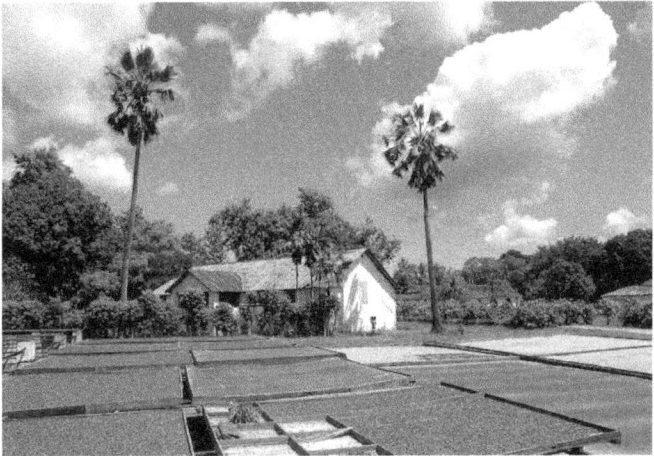

Beans dry in the Sun at a plantation in Madagascar, and microbes invisibly do their work

Microorganisms at work

Cacao fermentation is a multi-step process. Any compound microorganisms produced along the way that changes the taste of the beans will also change the taste of the final chocolate.

The first fermentation step may be familiar to home brewers, because it involves yeasts – some of them the same yeasts that ferment beer and wine. Just like the yeast in your favorite brew, yeast in a cacao fermentation produces alcohol by digesting the sugary pulp that clings to the beans.

This process generates fruity-tasting molecules called esters and floral-tasting fusel alcohols. These compounds soak into the beans and are later present in the finished chocolate.

As the pulp breaks down, oxygen enters the fermenting mass and the yeast population declines as oxygen-loving bacteria take over. These bacteria are known as acetic acid bacteria because they convert the alcohol generated by the yeast into acetic acid.

The acid soaks into the beans, causing biochemical changes. The sprouting plant dies. Fats agglomerate. Some enzymes break proteins down into smaller peptides, which become very "chocolatey"-smelling during the subsequent roasting stage. Other enzymes break apart the antioxidant polyphenol molecules, for which chocolate has gained renown as a superfood. As a result, contrary to its reputation, most chocolate contains very few polyphenols, or even none at all.

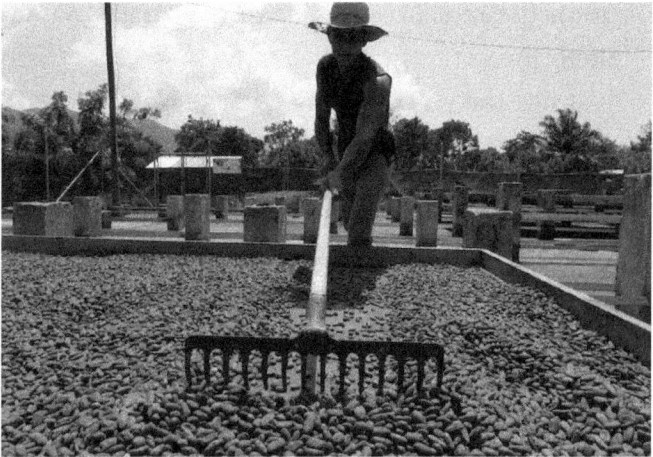

As the drying progresses, different microorganisms naturally emerge to do their job preparing the beans

All the reactions kicked off by acetic acid bacteria have a major impact on flavor. These acids encourage the degradation of heavily astringent, deep purple polyphenol molecules into milder-tasting, brown-colored chemicals called o-quinones. Here is where cacao beans turn from bitter-tasting to rich and nutty. This flavor transformation is accompanied by a color shift from reddish-purple to brown, and it is the reason the chocolate you're familiar with is brown and not purple.

Finally, as acid slowly evaporates and sugars are used up, other species – including filamentous fungi and spore-forming *Bacillus* bacteria – take over.

As vital as microbes are to the chocolate-making process, sometimes organisms can ruin a fermentation. An overgrowth of the spore-forming *Bacillus* bacteria is associated with compounds that lead to rancid, cheesy flavors.

Terroir of a place and its microbes

Cacao is a wild fermentation – farmers rely on natural microbes in the environment to create unique, local flavors. This phenomenon is known as "terroir": the characteristic flair imparted by a place. In the same way that grapes take on regional terroir, these wild microbes, combined with each farmer's particular process, confer terroir on beans fermented in each location.

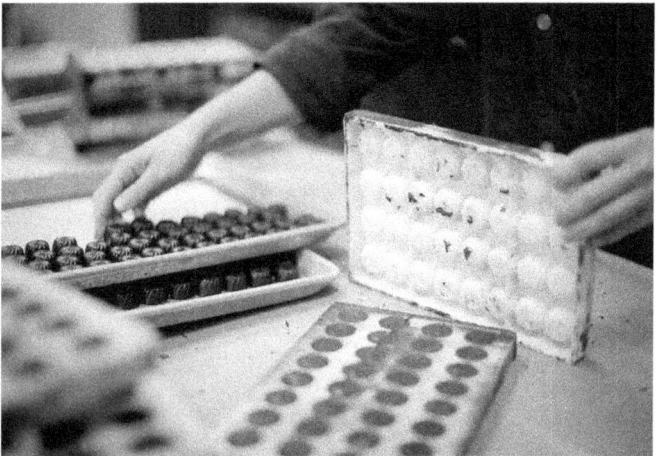

High-end chocolate-makers are choosy about their beans

Market demand for these fine, high-quality beans is growing. Makers of gourmet, small-batch chocolate hand-select beans based on their distinctive terroir in order to produce chocolate with an impressive range of flavor nuances.

If you've experienced chocolate only in the form of a bar you might grab near the grocery store checkout, you probably have little idea of the range and complexity that truly excellent chocolate can exhibit.

A bar from Akesson's Madagascar estate may be reminiscent of raspberries and apricots, while Canadian chocolate-maker Qantu's wild-fermented Peruvian bars taste like they've been soaked in Sauvignon Blanc. Yet in both cases, the bars contain nothing except cacao beans and some sugar.

This is the power of fermentation: to change, convert, transform. It takes the usual and make it unusual – thanks to the magic of microbes.

12. Chocolate chemistry

Whether it is enjoyed as creamy milk chocolate truffles, baked in a devilishly dark chocolate cake or even poured as hot cocoa, Americans on average consume almost 20 pounds (9 kilograms) of chocolate in a year. People have been enjoying chocolate for at least 4,000 years, starting with Mesoamericans who brewed a drink from the seeds of cacao trees. In the 16th and 17th centuries, both the trees and the beverage spread across the world, and chocolate today is a trillion-dollar global industry. I've conducted research on the volatile molecules that make chocolate taste good. I also developed and taught a very popular college course on the science of chocolate. Here are the answers to some of the most frequent questions I hear about this unique and complex food.

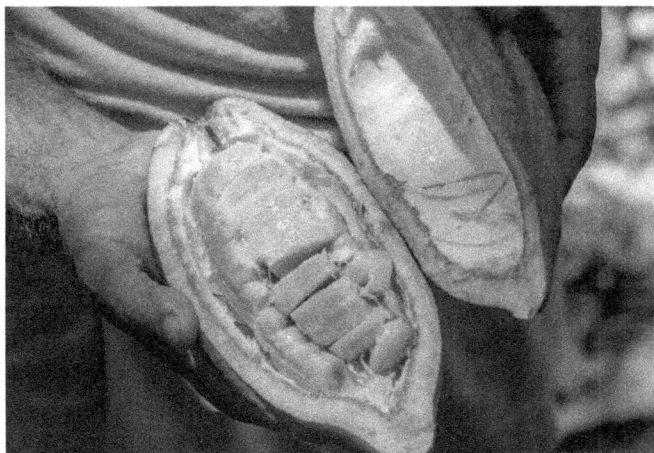

There's a lot of processing that happens between cacao beans in a pod and the chocolate at your table

How does chocolate get its characteristic flavor?

Chocolate starts out as a rather dull-tasting bean, packed into a pod that grows on a cacao tree. Developing the characteristic flavor of chocolate requires two key steps: fermentation and roasting.

Immediately after harvest, the beans are piled under leaves and left to ferment for several days. Bacteria create the chemicals, called precursors, needed for the next step: roasting.

The flavor you know as chocolate is formed during roasting by something chemists call the Maillard reaction. It requires two types of chemicals – sugar and protein – both of which are present in the fermented cacao beans. Roasting brings them together under high heat, which causes the sugar and protein to react and form that wonderful aroma.

Roasting is something of an art form. Different temperatures and times will produce different flavors. If you sample a few chocolate bars on the market, you will quickly realize that some companies roast at a much higher temperature than others. Lower temperatures maximize the floral and fruity notes, while higher temperatures create more caramel and coffee notes. Which is better is really a matter of personal preference.

Interestingly, the Maillard reaction is also what creates the flavor of freshly baked bread, roasted meat and coffee. The similarity between chocolate and coffee may seem fairly obvious, but bread and meat? The reason those foods all smell so different is that the flavor chemicals that get formed depend on the exact types of sugar and protein. Bread and chocolate contain different types, so even if you roasted them in exactly the same manner, you wouldn't get the same flavor. This specificity is part of the reason it's so hard to make a good artificial chocolate flavor.

How long can you store chocolate?

Once the beans are roasted, that wonderful aroma has been created. The longer you wait to consume it, the more of the volatile compounds responsible for the smell evaporate and the less flavor is left for you to enjoy. Generally, you have about a year to eat milk chocolate and two years for dark chocolate. It's not a good idea to store it in the refrigerator, because it picks up moisture and odors from the other things in there, but you can store it tightly sealed in the freezer.

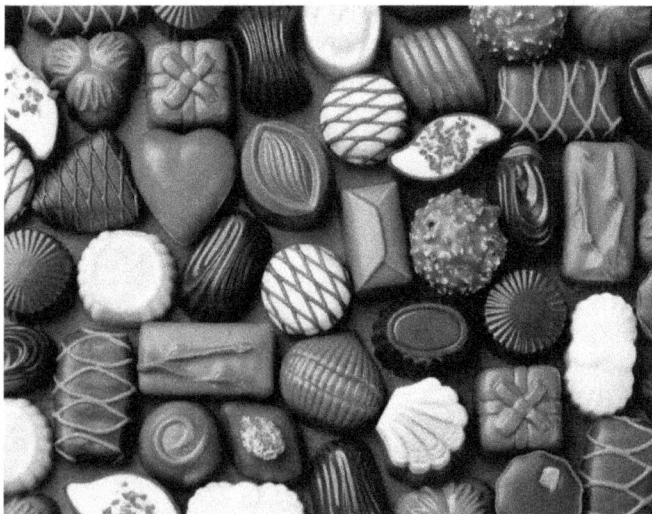

What's different about hot chocolate?

To make powdered hot chocolate, the beans are soaked in alkali to increase their pH before roasting. Raising the pH to be more basic helps make the powdered cocoa more soluble in water. But when the beans are at a higher pH during roasting, it changes the Maillard reaction so that different flavors are formed.

The flavor of hot chocolate is described by experts as a smooth and mellow flavor with earthy, woodsy notes, while regular chocolate flavor is sharp, with an almost citrus fruit finish.

What creates the texture of a chocolate bar?

Historically, chocolate was consumed as a drink because the ground beans are very gritty – far from the smooth, creamy texture people can create today.

After removing the shells and grinding the beans, modern chocolate makers add additional cocoa butter. Cocoa butter is the fat that occurs in the cacao beans. But there isn't enough fat naturally in the beans to make a smooth texture, so chocolate makers add extra.

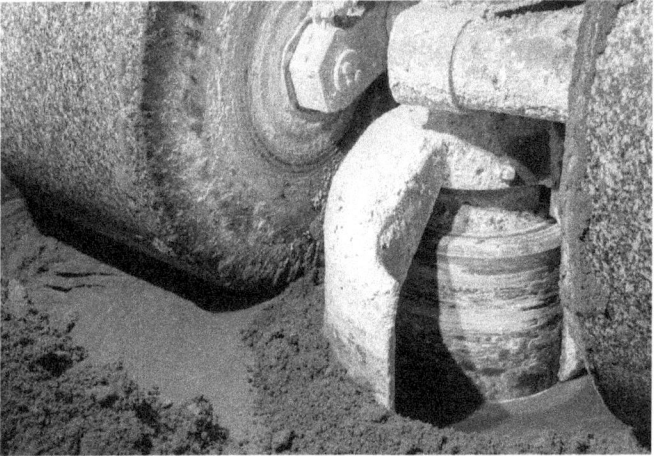

Machines can pulverize the beans to a very fine texture

Next the cacao beans and cocoa butter undergo a process called conching. When the process was first invented, it took a team of horses a week walking in a circle, pulling a large grinding stone, to pulverize the particles small enough. Today machines can do this grinding and mixing in about eight hours. This process creates a smooth texture, and also drives off some of the undesirable odors.

Why is chocolate so difficult to cook with?

The chocolate you buy in a store has been tempered. Tempering is a process of heating up the chocolate to just the right temperature during production, before letting it cool to a solid. This step is necessary because of the fat.

Cocoa butter's fat can naturally exist in six different crystal forms when it is a solid. Five of these are unstable and want to convert into the most stable, sixth form. Unfortunately, that sixth form is white in appearance, gritty in texture and is commonly called "bloom." If you see a chocolate bar with white spots on it, it has bloomed, which means the fat has rearranged itself into that sixth crystal form. It is still edible but doesn't taste as good.

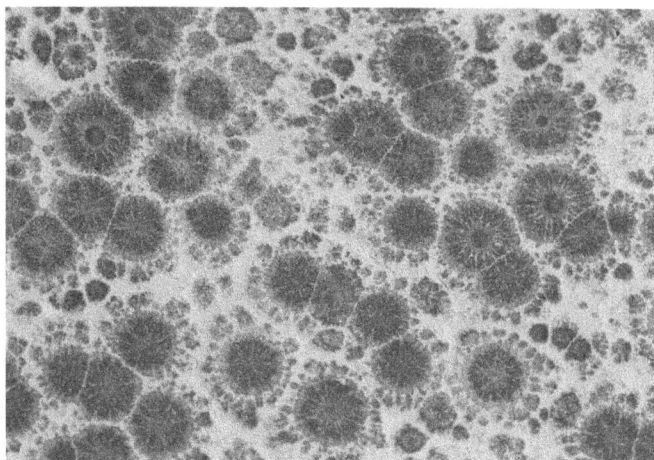

Careful chocolate prep tries to hold off the most stable – but undesirable – version of the fat in cocoa butter, which is called bloom.

You can't prevent bloom from happening, but you can slow it down by heating and cooling the chocolate through a series of temperature cycles. This process causes all the fat to crystallize into the second-most stable form. It takes a long time for this form to rearrange itself into the white, gritty sixth form.

When you melt chocolate at home, you break the temper. The day after you've created your confection, the chocolate usually blooms with an unattractive gray or white surface.

Is chocolate an aphrodisiac or antidepressant?

The short answer is, sorry, no. Eating chocolate may make you feel happier, but that's because it tastes so good, not because it is chemically changing your brain.

THE CHEMISTRY OF CHOCOLATE

IS CHOCOLATE AN APHRODISIAC?

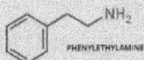

PHENYLETHYLAMINE

Phenylethylamine occurs naturally in the brain, and is often referred to as 'the love drug' due to its ability to produce feelings of well-being and contentment. It is also present in significant concentrations in chocolate, but since it is broken down after ingestion, it has been ruled out as causing a significant aphrodisiac effect.

Tryptophan is a chemical in the brain linked to the production of serotonin, the neurotransmitter that produces feelings of elation. It is present in chocolate, but only in small quantities, and it is unlikely that it causes any aphrodisiac effect.

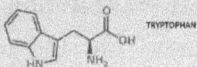

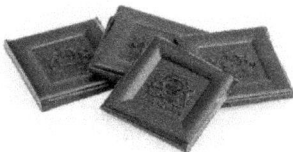

TRYPTOPHAN

WHY IS CHOCOLATE TOXIC TO DOGS?

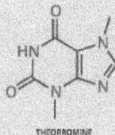

Theobromine is a mild stimulant, similar in effect to caffeine, found in chocolate. This compound is harmless to humans at the levels found in chocolate - a fatal dose would require eating tens of kilograms of milk chocolate!

In cats & dogs, theobromine has a much more potent effect; small doses can lead to vomiting & diarrhoea, whilst as little as 50g of dark chocolate could kill a small dog.

THEOBROMINE

13. It's a Wrap

We're at the end, which means you're about to go out into the wild as your very own chocolate expert. So thank you for joining me on this journey and letting me share the world's best chocolate with you. I just wanted to reiterate a couple of points that will help you go through that process to identify what the world's best chocolate is. So to start with, you need to care about the bean and what type of bean it is. And typically, we're talking about the Carrillo, the Trinitron. The National is being good. I did allude to before that there's the occasional Forestier bean. If you see someone actually proclaiming they use the Forestier, I'd give them a go and say that it's potentially a good thing. If they're using bad ones, they're just going to hide it away. Look at the packaging, then we should be looking for more than just words. You want to look for that transparency, not just where is it going by the country? Is it telling you about the plantation and things like that? You want it to be able to find out a little bit about it. Remember, single origin is a little bit dubious as a term. So we want to be looking for something like single estate or single plantation. But don't assume that blended beans are bad or blended chocolates are bad because that takes mastery to blend. Well, look for ethics. I can't stress that enough. You get onto a website, see what they're doing, look at what those genuine social enterprise and social support is, and I guess get out there and start trying chocolate. That's the that's the main way you discover what's good. And I do this myself. There is no magic formula to discovering what a good chocolate I know. The brands that I do with it are great. But otherwise, for me, I go out there, I see some clues on the packaging, what might be good, what might be bad. I know that chocolate from Madagascar is generally good from Venezuela, it's generally good, et cetera. But it's not until I buy it and try it that I know I bought a block of chocolate recently, a seventy five percent from Madagascar. I thought great Madagascan chocolate, lots of tangy red acidic fruit flavors. I got home and I tried it and it was really quite terrible. It had lots of different things on there about what made it good. So you never going to know until you try. Remember to look for being Jaber, which is typically a really good sign. If you're saying that, remember that the best comes from largely France and Italy. There are some other countries, but it's very, very rarely going to come from Belgium or Switzerland. So have your antennas out for that and go and enjoy your chocolate eating. And on my last little tip, always remember to eat that dark chocolate first because you're going to do a disservice to dark chocolate if you're having the milk first. I hope you've enjoyed your journey through chocolate. I hope you're going to go forth and eat the world's best chocolate.